How To Build Bigger Muscles Fast

309 Great Tips To Gain Muscle Mass

ADAM COLTON

Published by BizMove
www.bizmove.com

ISBN: 1979470901
ISBN- 978-1979470902

309 Great Tips To Gain Muscle Mass

Are you trying to get into better shape? Do you want to see some growth in your muscles? If you would like to see an increase in the size of your muscles, read the following ides. You will find helpful tips on increasing your muscle mass the right way.

1. Try doing real stairs instead of the stairs that your gym has. This can help change the perspective that you have for working out, give you an additional amount of motivation, burn more fat, and build more muscle. The additional scenery could also help you workout for a longer period of time.

2. Be sure that you add in as many reps and sets as possible as you workout. Fifteen lifts is a good number, with no more than a minute break between sets. This stimulates the release of lactic acid, which is a key component in muscle growth. When you constantly do this as you workout you help maximize the amount of muscles you build.

3. You need to know how many calories to eat per day in order to gain the muscle you want to gain. To determine your daily calorie intake you should multiple your weight by 15. The resulting number is

the number of calories your body needs to build muscle and burn as much fat as possible.

4. Make sure you are eating enough food to support new muscle growth. Many people struggle with not eating enough to support the kind of growth they are trying to achieve. If you are trying to lose weight and build muscle at the same time, make sure you are eating protein rich foods to help with muscle growth.

5. Aim to maintain a journal when following a workout regimen. Jot down the exercises that you do, the number of sets and reps you do, and anything else concerning your workout. You should write down how much rest you get each night and even how you feel during workouts. Writing down everything that you can allows you to better keep track of how you are doing every single week.

6. You should try to make use of chains and bands in your weight workouts. These things add a type of resistance that is referred to as LVRT. This gives you a greater amount of tension because your range of motion is increasing in a single movement, which can lead to more muscle growth.

7. Perform your lifting regimen every other day. After a vigorous workout, the protein synthesis process

can take up to 48 hours to complete. In other words, your body builds muscle for up to two-day post-workout, and working out while your body is still recovering may undo your hard work. Enjoy the day of rest--it will help to maximize your results.

8. Consider making use of tri-sets in your workout plan. These sets involve doing three exercises simultaneously, and you do these exercises all together without any form of rest. Tri-sets is an excellent method of shocking a plateaued muscle that needs to wake up in order for it to grow in size.

9. When attempting to grow muscle mass, utilize the buddy system method. This involves you and your partner pushing each other in a different manner. One person competes a set, and then he or she passes the dumbbells or bar to the other person. Except for the amount of time that you are waiting on your partner to finish a set, you do not rest.

10.   You have an overwhelming selection of workout machines or programs for you to try. It is sometimes easy to forget that not all methods are effective for all goals or all athletes.

11.   Building muscles it's easily accomplished when you customize a routine and stick with it. There are many options for building muscles. Do your

research and investigate the best workout tools and techniques to get the look that you want. You may even have a workout friend that can help you increase your result.

12.   Watch your form when you are working out. Maintaining poor form is the surest way to harm your body, meaning that you have to take time off from your exercise routine and have no chance of seeing the results that you are looking for. Talk to a trainer if you are not sure about your form, and make sure that you get it right before you even begin doing repetitions.

13.   Always try to eat after your workouts. As soon as you are done working out, go have something to eat. It does not have to be a full meal. It can be as easy as a glass of juice or soy protein. This will help your muscles properly recover from the workout.

14.   If you are a beginner at building muscle, try to focus your lifting routine so that you can do between 8 and 12 repetitions of each exercise. If you are able to do more, then you probably are not lifting a heavy enough load. By giving yourself a goal, you will also help to ensure that you continue working out until you reach the point of fatigue.

15.   While whole foods are the best way to get your calories in general, a protein shake after your workout might actually be easier for your body to digest and process. A quick shot of protein after a workout gives your body the building blocks to keep adding muscle, instead of using existing muscle to replenish its energy reserves.

16.   To gain that lean muscle mass, be sure to use free weights. These have been proven to work better than cables and machines for building lean muscle. Free weights allow you to use many different muscles as you lift. This way, you will be stimulating added muscle growth by working the extra muscles.

17.   Try to consume some carbohydrates and proteins prior to going to sleep. The calories that you obtain will cause your body to reduce the rate at which it breaks down proteins while you are sleeping. Eating a small portion of cheese and a fruit is a great way to do this. You should also eat something soon after you wake up.

18.   Remember the "big three," and include these exercises in your routine. Squats, dead lifts and bench presses all build muscle mass quickly. These types of exercises help add bulk in addition to strengthening and conditioning your body. It's

important to tailor your exercises to include variations of these regularly.

19.   A great way to build muscle is to pay close attention to nutrition, and eat a good amount of protein and carbohydrates. By eating every two hours, and ensuring you get no less than 1.5 grams of protein for each pound of your own weight and no less than 2 grams of carbohydrates per pound. You will have the nutritional tools necessary to build muscle.

20.   Use visualization exercises to picture what you need to do to reach your goals. Having vague, undefined goals with no real sense of how to accomplish them is a sure road to failure. Picture yourself sticking to your workout routine and visualize what you will look like in the future. This will keep you motivated.

21.   Provide your body with plenty of the right fuel on exercise days. Fuel up for your exercise session by taking in some calories an hour before heading to the gym. This does not mean that you should eat too much, but eat more than you would on a day that you would not work out.

22.   When training, high reps and a good number of sets will show the best results. Do fifteen lifts at the

minimum with a break of a minute or less in between. By doing this, you are letting your lactic acids flow, which in turn, helps muscle growth. Doing this several times a session can help vastly.

23.   Only workout your abs muscles two to three times per week. Many people make the mistake of doing abdominal exercises daily. This does not give the muscles enough time to recover and can ultimately limit their growth and could cause your body to become injured. Working out two to three times per week is sufficient to get lean abs.

24.   Always use your own intuition when working out. Although planning out your workouts ahead is good for making sure that you stay accountable, sometimes you can't always stick to this schedule. For example, you might not be ready for another quad session after your last session left you exhausted. On the other hand, your arms could be well rested after a good workout just a few days ago. Listen to what your body tells you, and follow it.

25.   Remember that it is never a good idea to use the scale to determine your progress when you are trying to build muscle. If you find that your scale is increasing in numbers, remember that you just might be losing fat while gaining muscle. Since muscle weighs more than fat, this is a familiar site

for many who are trying to do both at the same time. Gauge your results by what you see in the mirror rather than what you see on the scale.

26.   It is difficult to lose weight and build muscle at the same time. You have to have a high-protein diet to support your muscle growth, but reduce your fat intake at the same time. Eat foods that are high in protein and low in fat and refined carbohydrates to reduce weight and gain muscle at the same time.

27.   Remember to go to the gym with a friend when you are working on building up your muscles. If you try to do so alone, it is possible that you put yourself into a difficult situation, especially when using free weights. This can lead to serious injuries or lesions.

28.   Keep good records. Have a workout diary, which notes the exercises in your workout routine, and how many reps and sets you perform. This not only helps to keep your workouts organized, but you can see your progress. This is inspiring, especially at first when progress is made rapidly. You can see how far you have come and set goals.

29.   Do not overlook the importance of rest in muscle growth. Believe it or not, growth actually occurs during rest, so if you are not getting enough

of it, your muscled will not grow or be adequately conditioned. Working out stimulates muscles, and during rest your body gets to work at building the muscles. You need to understand this process and factor rest into your muscle conditioning or building routine.

30.   Make sure you are eating enough. Even if you are trying to lose weight while you build muscle, it is important that you are consuming sufficient calories. When your body is deprived of its fuel, it will be difficult to build muscle. An ideal diet for muscle gain is high in protein and low in fat and refined (processed) carbohydrates.

31.   Focus on one thing at a time. If you want to build mass, you should concentrate on mass building exercises rather than developing your cardio. Working on your cardio will help you develop other parts of your body and might slow down the building of your muscles if it becomes the focus of your training.

32.   You will be able to build muscle faster if you take breaks between workout, days in contrast to working out every day. The reason for this is that muscles heal and grow while you are resting, and not while you are exercising. Create a workout

routine that alternates between workout and rest days.

33.   It is important to eat foods and meals with carbohydrates after your workout and on your rest days. This will help you to rebuild and grow your muscles faster. The reason for this is that consuming carbohydrates causes the production of insulin in your body which in turn slows down the rate at which your body breaks down proteins. Even something as simple as a banana or a peanut butter sandwich will help.

34.   Regardless of how frequent or intense your workout sessions are, if you are not eating sufficiently, your body will not have enough proteins to build muscle. It is therefore critical to eat meals often. You should strive to consume at least 20 grams of protein every three hours. In addition, it is more important to eat often rather than to eat large portions.

35.   It is important to get a sufficient amount of sleep and rest after your workout sessions. A significant amount of muscle recovery and repair occurs while you are sleeping. Not getting an adequate amount of sleep can delay your results, and also be dangerous. Working out again without proper recuperation can cause injury or illness.

36.   Always include the "big three" exercises in your training schedule. These mass building exercises include dead lifts, bench presses and squats. These exercise add muscle mass, improve balance, and make your body stronger and more agile. Add variations of these exercises to your usual workouts.

37.   You should completely exert yourself when performing weight lifting exercises in order to maximize your muscle gain results. Do this by forcing yourself to keep doing one more repetition until you absolutely cannot. This sends a clear signal to your body that you need more muscle. Remember to get help from a spotter so that you do not suddenly drop the weight when you are finished.

38.   Use visualization exercises to picture what you need to do to reach your goals. Having vague, undefined goals with no real sense of how to accomplish them is a sure road to failure. Picture yourself sticking to your workout routine and visualize what you will look like in the future. This will keep you motivated.

39.   Remember to go to the gym with a friend when you are working on building up your muscles. If you try to do so alone, it is possible that you put

yourself into a difficult situation, especially when using free weights. This can lead to serious injuries or lesions.

40.   It is OK to take a few short-cuts when weight lifting. While you are trying to finish some extra reps, you can use only a little bit of your body if it will help you get it done. This will help you to increase how much you are working out. You just cannot constantly fudge and get the desired results. Keep a controlled rep speed. Don't let your reps get sloppy.

41.   Consider using strip sets when working out. This involves doing as many reps of a weight as you can, and after doing this, reducing the weight by up to twenty to thirty percent and going to failure again. This method can help you grow those stubborn muscles that just won't grow anymore.

42.   Take a break occasionally, your body needs some time to recover from your workouts so that it has the opportunity to regrow muscle tissue. This is why the most effective method for building muscle is to work out for a couple of days and then take a day off.

43.   You should monitor your intake of carbohydrates. If your diet is too poor in carbs,

your muscles will be used to fuel your body while you exercise. You should be eating between two and three grams of carbs for each pound of your weight every day. Make sure you are getting your carbs from healthy aliments.

44.   Try switching the grip for your back. Grip the weight bar with a staged or mixed grip position when performing deadlifts and rack pulls, to achieve a varied workout and better overall results. A staggered grip will help you twist the bar in a singular direction, while at the same time, your underhand twists the bar in another direction. This helps you keep the bar steady, rather than having it roll all over the place.

45.   Complete those exercises that work more than one muscle group first, and then work on the ones that require the use of an isolated muscle. Doing this will allow you to complete the exercises that use the most energy first, while you are still feeling fresh and energetic. You will complete a more effective workout and put focus on working your entire body, rather than just one muscle group.

46.   If you are a beginner at building muscle, try to focus your lifting routine so that you can do between 8 and 12 repetitions of each exercise. If you are able to do more, then you probably are not

lifting a heavy enough load. By giving yourself a goal, you will also help to ensure that you continue working out until you reach the point of fatigue.

47.   Train at least three times per week. You need at least three training sessions every week if you want to see significant muscle growth. If you are really new at weight training, this can be reduced to two at the start; however, you should increase the number of sessions per week as soon as you are able. If you already have some experience with strength training, you can add more sessions as well.

48.   Refrain from performing both strength training and cardiovascular exercises, if your goal is to build muscle, and not necessarily to improve overall fitness. The reason for this is that these two kinds of exercises cause your body to respond in contradictory ways. Focusing strictly on building muscle will help you to maximize your results.

49.   Lifting heavy weights is productive for many parts of the body, but you should avoid lifting extreme amounts of weight when you are working out by performing neck work, dips and split squats. If the exercise puts you in a joint position that is unfavorable, keep the weight limit to a reasonable level.

50.   You should consider getting a personal trainer. A personal trainer is trained in what specific exercises will help you build muscle. Your personal trainer will also help you with a variety of tips including things like what you should be eating as well as supplement advice. In addition to this, your personal trainer will push you when you need to pushed to go that extra mile to help you build your muscles.

51.   If you are on a program to build muscle, try losing any excess weight you are carrying first. You must consume fewer calories than you burn. Any activity such as mowing the lawn, bike riding or swimming will create a caloric deficit. As you lose weight, you will begin to see your muscles appear. Then it's time to work them!

52.   Performing squats is essential for lifting routines. The squat incorporates many different muscle groups. Not only are your glute and quad muscles activated, but your lower back, hamstrings, core, and shoulders are also utilized. People who do squats regularly have been proven to have more muscle mass than those who do not.

53.   It is important to stay hydrated when building muscle. Failing to maintain proper hydration leaves you susceptible to injury. Furthermore, staying

hydrated makes it much easier to build and maintain your muscle mass.

54.   Use compound exercises to more efficiently add mass to your muscles. Exercises that target a single muscle group are fine later on, but when you are trying to bulk up in general, it's best to hit as many muscle groups as you can simultaneously. Pull-ups, chin-ups, squats, deadlifts and bench presses are all great exercises that work several muscle groups.

55.   Set goals that you can realistically achieve. Although you would like to squat several hundred pounds in only a month, this is just not possible, and you are likely to injure yourself. After finding your baseline strength, attempt to modestly improve every routine. Don't be surprised if you occasionally blow past short-term goals. Use this as encouragement to keep working out.

56.   When you work out, you should always be counting how many push ups or squats you are doing. Keeping track of your performance is a good way to know if you are actually progressing. With time, you should do your best to increase the number of sets you can do.

57.   Consider using caffeine on a limited basis as a benefit to bodybuilding. Metabolism can be

increased by drinking a cup of coffee in the morning, and caffeine can increase overall calorie burn. The intensity of workout routines can be increased by the stimulant, and caffeine can provide energy after a hard workout.

58.   Try to find a friend to workout with. By having someone there, you will have someone who can push your limits a bit when you need it. This is especially nice if your workout buddy is at the same level that you are. Having a friend to workout with is also helps since certain weightlifting exercises do require a spotter.

59.   Be sure that you are warming up before each workout. If you don't warm up properly, you are at risk of injuring a muscle or tendon and ending your workouts for a long period of time. Warm up by doing some cardio exercise and lifting some light weights. Your body will thank you!

60.   When you are starting your workout, make sure that you set reasonable goals. If your goals are unreachable, you are setting yourself up to fall short of the accomplishments that you desire, which can be devastating. Analyze what you can and cannot do and leverage off of this information before you set your goals.

61.   Once in a while, you should replace your usual training routine by a completely different workout. Go out for a jog or head out to the local swimming pool, for instance. You will notice how much easier these activities have become for you, and this will help you stay motivated.

62.   Many women who want to build lean muscle mass sometimes do too much cardio. After about a half hour of cardio, your body will turn to muscle for energy, causing you to lose what you've worked so hard for! By keeping the cardio to 20-25 minutes, you can keep your lean muscle intact!

63.   If you would like to build more muscle mass, try to do less repetitions of heaver weights. You will need to increase your weight gradually and strive to lift the heaviest that you possibly can for a minimum of five repetitions. When you can life for five repetitions, it is time to increase weights.

64.   Don't keep your routine the same all the time. Your muscles will soon get accustomed to your workouts and you will cease to see positive results. Engage in different exercises each time you workout to ensure you work different groups each time. This will keep you motivated by staving off boredom.

65.   Genetics are going to play a role in the amount of muscle building success that you see. If your family has not provided you with the right genetics to have the body that you dream of, you may have to work doubly as hard to see any results. That does not mean it is impossible, it just means more hard work.

66.   If you want to make sure that you have the very best muscle growth you can, it is vital you perform compound exercises. These particular exercises will allow you to exercise several muscle groups in each lift. For example, a bench press will utilize shoulder, tricep and chest muscles all at once.

67.   Eat plenty of carbs. If your body runs short on glucose after hard workouts, your body will use muscle tissue for protein and carbohydrates, undoing your hard work. Stay away from low-carb diets, and eat an appropriate amount of carbs given the intensity of your workouts--possibly a couple of grams of carbs per pound of body weight each day.

68.   Spread your workouts out so that you are only lifting weights every other day. Spend one day working out your entire body, and then use the next day to rest. Your muscles will grow while you rest, not while you are working out. Even though it

might feel like you are doing nothing on your days off, your body is still working hard.

69.   Fill up on carbohydrates after a workout. It has been proven that if you do this, on the days that you are not going to work out, you will be rebuilding your muscles faster. Eating carbs after a workout increases insulin levels, which slows down the rate that your body breaks down protein.

70.   Pay attention to your body fat and measure it on a regular basis. Try not to be discouraged if there is not significant weight loss when building muscle, because your weight might not change much using a weight and muscle building routine. Your body fat is a better measure of your overall health as opposed to weight.

71.   Performing squats is essential for lifting routines. The squat incorporates many different muscle groups. Not only are your glute and quad muscles activated, but your lower back, hamstrings, core, and shoulders are also utilized. People who do squats regularly have been proven to have more muscle mass than those who do not.

72.   Muscle building is a very interesting activity, but it is one that requires preparation and knowledge to avoid injury. Don't just run to the gym thinking that

you can learn as you go. Either go together with an experienced friend or do some research beforehand to know what to expect.

73.   Try to eat every 3-4 hours. If you don't eat frequently enough, you can slow down the rate at which your body creates new proteins, which create muscle tissue. Divide the total number of calories you need in a day by 6, and try to shoot for 6 mini-meals spread out over the course of the day.

74.   Whenever you are working out in order to build muscles, you should have a well-defined goal in mind. Aim to increase the number of reps you do, the maximum weight that you use, or the overall length of your workout. In order to really improve your muscles, rather than simply exercise them, you need to keep them constantly challenged.

75.   Get better at bicep curling. You only get half the benefit you could get from a normal bicep curl, as you likely don't move the bar beyond the parallel point during the "up" part of the exercise. The strongest portion of bicep curls is the top portion. You can solve this problem by doing barbell curls while sitting down.

76.   When building muscle, many people make the mistake of over training. When you go to the gym,

exercise as hard as possible and take short breaks. Do not do your workouts for more than 60 minutes for best results. Go in, workout, and get out to give your muscles time to recover.

77.   Your diet is as important as your workout when building muscle mass. Specific nutrients are required for your body to build muscle. There have been studies done that show drinking protein shakes after a workout is beneficial for muscle fiber rebuilding.

78.   Consider creatine supplementation. This could give you the push you need to be able to drive through a workout and give it your all. Make sure that you are careful if you are taking any type of supplement. Use these products in accordance with your body size and only as directed.

79.   Always do 10 minutes of stretching prior to lifting weights. This will help to prevent injury by warming up your muscles before they are asked to lift a heavy load. This routine can also help you to avoid normal everyday injuries caused by tight, inflexible muscles. This will allow you to continue your exercise plan unhindered.

80.   Your top three exercises will be a squat, deadlift and bench press. There is a good reason these

exercises are thought of as the cornerstone of good bodybuilding. They have proven to increase strength, add bulk to muscles, and improve your general level of conditioning. Include these three in some way at each workout.

81.   Have protein before starting a workout. Whether you have a sandwich with about 4 ounces of lunch meat, a protein bar or a shake, it's important to remember that protein synthesis is what is important for building muscle. Have your protein about half an hour to an hour before starting a workout for best results.

82.   Eating some meat can help your muscles grow. A good protein target is one gram of protein per pound of mass. Doing this will assist you in storing more protein. The greater amount of protein that you consume, the larger your muscles will get. Eventually, your muscles will achieve the size that you've been wanting.

83.   Do not attempt extreme cardio training with weight training. Done within reason, this combo can be truly beneficial for your health, but when done in extreme fashions can contradict one another minimizing the results that you see from either one of them. Pick one to focus on and stay committed to working on it regularly.

84.   If you are on a program to build muscle, try losing any excess weight you are carrying first. You must consume fewer calories than you burn. Any activity such as mowing the lawn, bike riding or swimming will create a caloric deficit. As you lose weight, you will begin to see your muscles appear. Then it's time to work them!

85.   Fill up on carbohydrates after a workout. It has been proven that if you do this, on the days that you are not going to work out, you will be rebuilding your muscles faster. Eating carbs after a workout increases insulin levels, which slows down the rate that your body breaks down protein.

86.   As you become more experienced in working out, it's very important that you make sure to adjust the amount of weight you lift. Once you get stronger, you are either going to have to increase your weight or your reps in order to get that pump you need for achieving additional muscle growth. Try to increase gradually the amount of weight you lift to ensure that you don't overexert yourself.

87.   When beginning a muscle-building program, lots of people increase the amount of protein they consume too much too soon. Doing so may lead to excessive calorie consumption, which might then

cause you to gain weight in the form of body fat. Increase protein intake slowly so your body can transform it into muscle well.

88.   Make sure that you are incorporating some full body workouts in your muscle building routine. Muscles support each other, so if you work them all you will have a better chance of seeing the best results. You might even see some health problems if all of your workouts consist of only working on a few isolated muscles.

89.   Performing squats is essential for lifting routines. The squat incorporates many different muscle groups. Not only are your glute and quad muscles activated, but your lower back, hamstrings, core, and shoulders are also utilized. People who do squats regularly have been proven to have more muscle mass than those who do not.

90.   A good muscle building program will increase your strength. Ultimately, you should see an advancement in the amount of weight you are able to lift. If you are new to weight lifting, you should see an increase of approximately 5% in the weight you can lift every other workout session. You need to reassess your program if your progress is slower than this. If you sense you have not gained strength

since your last workout, you may not have allowed yourself sufficient recovery time.

91.   Your workout routine always needs goals, so set a new goal as soon as you have achieved an old one. Reaching a goal feels great, and you deserve to feel proud of your accomplishment. Just remember that building muscle is a process that you can keep working at indefinitely, as long as you have a fresh goal to aim for.

92.   You need to be mindful of your caloric intake, if you want to build muscle. You want to only consume food that provides healthy calories for muscle building while avoiding foods that are bad for you. If you eat a poor diet, you will fail to build muscle and will become fat.

93.   If your training regimen has reached four days weekly, then try to avoid having more than one pair of consecutive down days. Your body will build and recover better with the down days spread out. If your life and schedule make this impossible, do not lose any sleep over it though, as you are still working out four days a week.

94.   Free weights are better for building muscle mass than machines. Machines have their uses, but force the body into strict motions. With free weights, you

can lift more and with greater range of motion. They also help to improve your body's balance, of which machines are incapable. In addition, if you workout at home, free weights are less expensive and take up a smaller footprint than machines.

95.   Consider employing the services of a personal trainer. An experienced personal training can use their expertise to create a tailor-made workout plan for you to follow, which will help you to build your muscles quickly and safely. If you continue to work out without professional guidance, it could take you much longer to get the physique that you desire.

96.   Obtaining a workout partner can drastically improve your muscle-building results. Your partner can be a valuable source of motivation for sticking to your workout session, and pushing you to maximize your efforts while you work out. Having a reliable partner to work out with can also help keep you safe because you will always have a spotter.

97.   Many trainers will advise you to change your workout routine every few months. You should however keep in mind that this is not necessary. If the routine that you are using is providing excellent results, then you should stick with it! Change your routine only if it is not giving you the results that

you seek, or if you feel that you have gained most of the benefits from it.

98.   Don't try to focus on both cardio and strength at the same time. This is not to say you should not perform cardiovascular exercises when you are attempting to build muscle. In fact, cardio is an important part of physical fitness. However, you should not heavily train cardio, such as preparing for a marathon, if you are trying to focus on building muscle. The two types of exercises can conflict, minimizing effectiveness on both fronts.

99.   If you are trying to build muscle mass, it is important to eat calorie-dense food at the right time. The best time to eat your heaviest meal of the day is after you have completed your muscle-building workout session. It is at this time that the energy demands of your body are at peak levels since your body needs the nutrition to repair and build muscles. If you continue to eat some more calorie-dense food every couple of hours, you will provide an opportunity for your body to add even more muscle mass.

100.   In order to successfully gain muscle, it is important to have a strategy, and a plan to execute that strategy. There are various resources that you can utilize to determine which strength-training

exercises your plan will incorporate. You should also set a schedule that is easy to follow, and will not overwhelm you. Go over your plan with a professional trainer to make certain that it can fulfill your goals.

101.   Even though you might believe lifting heavy weights is the best method of building muscle, this isn't always the case. Lifting light weight is also very important when it comes to building muscle. Lifting different amounts of weight work different muscle fibers, which can help you ensure that your muscle gain is of higher quality.

102.   Consuming a sufficient amount of protein is a significant factor in building muscle. An excellent method of consuming an adequate amount of protein is by making use of supplements, such as protein shakes. Such beverages are especially useful following exercise and just prior to bedtime. To ensure that you shed pounds while building muscle, use a supplement daily. If you are looking to build both mass and muscle, drink up to three per day.

103.   Do not skimp on the amount of sleep you get. The process of building and repairing your muscles happens while you sleep, and without adequate recovery, you run the risk of hurting yourself during

workouts. Get 7-9 hours of sleep each night to maximize the benefits of the exercises you perform.

104.   You need to drink at least 4 liters of water every day if you want your muscles to grow. The body needs water to function properly but muscles need water to be able to rebuild after a workout and to grow in size. Drinking water is easy if you carry a water bottle with you everywhere you go.

105.   When doing a workout it is important to focus on only one exercise per body part when doing a full-body workout. This will help to ensure that you are maximizing your workout and not risking an injury. This will also help you to focus on your breathing and doing the exercises properly.

106.   Make sure that you select the best weight for yourself when doing lifting exercises. Research has proven that doing six to twelve reps at around seventy to eighty percent of your maximum for one rep, will give you the best combination of both volume and load. This can stimulate additional muscle growth.

107.   Change up your workouts. Research has proven that varying your reps, intensity, and exercises are the best combination for increasing muscle mass. Our bodies are very good at adapting to exercises,

and they have to be shocked by changing up the exercises in order to achieve the most optimum growth.

108.   Try to do bench presses and squats in the same manner that you do deadlifts, which is from a complete stop. Utilize bench and squat movements in the power rack, and allow the safety bars to be set at a certain point where this bar is at the bottom of these moves. You need to let the bar settle on this point. This helps you to remove any elastic tension, which assists you in increasing your strength.

109.   Your workout routine always needs goals, so set a new goal as soon as you have achieved an old one. Reaching a goal feels great, and you deserve to feel proud of your accomplishment. Just remember that building muscle is a process that you can keep working at indefinitely, as long as you have a fresh goal to aim for.

110.   Keep track of the time that it takes you to complete your workouts. A lot of people put their focus on the amount of weight they're lifting, their reps, and the amount of rest that they get. However, few people focus on the total amount of time that they work out. By focusing on achieving a shorter workout time by doing the same amount of work,

you can shorten the amount of time spent in the gym and maximize the effectiveness of your workout.

111.   If you would like to build more muscle mass, try to do less repetitions of heaver weights. You will need to increase your weight gradually and strive to lift the heaviest that you possibly can for a minimum of five repetitions. When you can life for five repetitions, it is time to increase weights.

112.   Genetics are one of the most important factors in building muscle mass. There is not much you can change about your interior genetics that shape your body, but you can improve the way you look by becoming more tone. Some of us just do not have the bodies that will have large muscles, so accept that and strive for better tone.

113.   Keep your protein intake high to increase muscle mass. Protein is the building block that muscles are made of. Lack of protein makes increasing muscle mass difficult. Try to eat healthy, lean proteins in two of the three major meals and one or two of your snacks every day.

114.   When trying to build muscle mass quickly, smaller is better. Smaller sets with more weight will add muscle more quickly than longer sets. Between

8-12 repetitions for each set is about the ideal. Give your body plenty of rest between workout routines to allow the body to heal. Muscle is built as the muscles heal.

115.   If you really want to start gaining muscle, consider getting a trainer. A trainer is an expert and has likely been where you are now. Ask a trainer about what kind of exercises are best, what kind of diet you should have and how often you should be at the gym. Trainers can be a great source of information and motivation so you can meet your own muscle building goals.

116.   In order to build muscle, it is important to maintain detailed records of your progress, and how you got there. By taking the time to jot down a few notes on the exercises and repetitions performed in each workout session, you will be able to consistently build upon what you have already done, and continue to grow stronger and build more muscle.

117.   Make sure that you select the best weight for yourself when doing lifting exercises. Research has proven that doing six to twelve reps at around seventy to eighty percent of your maximum for one rep, will give you the best combination of both

volume and load. This can stimulate additional muscle growth.

118.   Keep in mind that muscles don't grow while you're working out; they grow during the resting period when they feel sore. For this reason, it's most efficient to alternate workout days to give your muscles time to rest and grow. Working out heavily every single day will just wear your muscles down.

119.   Try training just one side of your body. By doing this, you are able to utilize an additional amount of your body's muscle fibers, which can cause you to increase your strength and muscle size a lot more effectively. Examples of this type of training include single-leg presses, single-arm overhead presses, and one-arm pulldowns.

120.   Make sure that your caloric intake, overall, is as high as it needs to be. There are a lot of tools online that can assist you in finding out how many calories you need to what you want to gain. Use these calculators, and alter your diet to get plenty of carbs, protein, and other vital nutrients to help build your muscles.

121.   Make sure that your diet has enough protein when you are trying to build muscle mass. The

maximum amount of protein intake you need is about one gram of protein for every pound of your body weight on a daily basis. Slightly more or less protein does not matter too much, but you do need to intake as much as possible.

122.   A frustrating part of muscle building is that some muscle groups show immediate results, while others take longer to develop. To target these areas, try using a fill set. These brief sets of 25-30 rep exercises can target those problem groups if it's done at least a couple days following your last rough workout.

123.   Volume is an important component of muscle growth. An excellent method of building muscle is by utilizing German Volume Training. This type of training instructs you to perform ten sets of ten reps for just one exercise. It's ideal that this exercise is a compound one in order to achieve the most growth.

124.   Keep protein going into your body both before and after a workout for maximum muscle building effects. About half an hour to an hour before working out, make sure to consume a good 20 grams of protein. This can easily be accommodated with a couple of glasses of milk or protein shake.

Do the same an hour after your work out also, and you will enhance your muscle-building efforts!

125.   Measure body fat, not body weight. Do not get discouraged if you are attempting to build muscle and you do not see a change in your weight. You can lose fat while you gain muscle, resulting in a weight that does not change. A better indicator is measuring your body fat. If your weight is holding steady (or even increasing) while your fat levels are dropping - you are gaining muscle.

126.   To build bigger muscles, you should always eat as soon as you get up in the morning. An early breakfast prevents your body from breaking down muscle tissue for energy, which will simply slow down your progress. Choose high-protein foods, and ensure you also eat plenty of carbs at breakfast.

127.   Aim for a high number of reps with medium-intensity weight when you train. For each individual exercise you do, try to do a set of 10 to 15 reps, resting less than one minute in between each set. This causes lactic acid to build up in your muscles, which makes you "feel the burn" while stimulating growth.

128.   Are you trying to add muscle mass to your body? If you are eating calorie-dense foods and are

performing muscle build workouts but are still not seeing the results that you desire, you might want to consider adding creatine supplements to boost the growth of your muscles. Creatine aids in building muscle mass. Not only is this supplement popular with many professional bodybuilders, it is also popular with many elite athletes in other sports.

129.   Stay active on your rest days. Being active increases your blood flow, and will help you to recover more quickly. The activity can be as simple as going for a walk. You can also go swimming, biking, or even get a massage. Engaging in these kinds of activities is significantly more effective than simply lying in bed all day.

130.   Crank up some music. Research has shown that listening to music you love while you are lifting can help you do more reps than not listening to any music at all or not listening to the music that you like. In addition, having headphones can help distract you from having a conversation with others that will defer your workout.

131.   Lifting heavy weights is productive for many parts of the body, but you should avoid lifting extreme amounts of weight when you are working out by performing neck work, dips and split squats. If the exercise puts you in a joint position that is

unfavorable, keep the weight limit to a reasonable level.

132.   Make sure to get an ample amount of sleep each night. Your muscles need time to repair themselves after you strain them during weight lifting sessions. If you do not allow the muscles to rest enough, it can lessen the results that you see from your weight lifting efforts dramatically.

133.   Don't bother lifting for more than an hour at a time. Your body will begin to produce cortisol, due to the stress it's enduring, if you push beyond sixty minutes. Cortisol has been shown to block testosterone, reducing the results you achieve. Making sure that workouts are less than an hour helps you to get the best results.

134.   Utilize a power rack in order to prevent a barbell from crushing you while doing a large squat. Lots of squat racks contain pins that can be set below the maximum squatting depth. If you reach failure on a rep, you can just allow the weight to drop onto these safety pins. Therefore, you don't have to worry about lifting more than you are capable of.

135.   Allow yourself to eat some ice cream. Studies have shown that eating one bowl of any type of ice cream that you like about two hours after a workout

does some good. It will trigger the surge of insulin in your body better than many other foods will, and it will taste good too!

136.   On the days after your workouts, it's best to rest and eat a lot of carbohydrates. This helps your body to build muscle and recover from expending energy during the workout. That way, you'll see the biggest muscle growth possible from the workout you did. Pasta, peanut butter sandwiches, and similar foods are great for this.

137.   In order to avoid burnout you should change up your routine from time to time. This means that you don't want to follow the exact same exercise plan for more than 8 consecutive weeks. Not only does this keep things interesting, it also helps your body continue to grow.

138.   Volume is an important component of muscle growth. An excellent method of building muscle is by utilizing German Volume Training. This type of training instructs you to perform ten sets of ten reps for just one exercise. It's ideal that this exercise is a compound one in order to achieve the most growth.

139.   Have reasonable and realistic expectations for yourself. The best hard bodies are the result of a lot

of time and effort, so don't expect to look like a body building world champion after a week or two of working out. Have a solid and healthy plan and dedicate yourself to it over a period of time. You will see results and doing it in a healthy and calculated manner will be much healthier for you.

140.   Try to eat every 3-4 hours. If you don't eat frequently enough, you can slow down the rate at which your body creates new proteins, which create muscle tissue. Divide the total number of calories you need in a day by 6, and try to shoot for 6 mini-meals spread out over the course of the day.

141.   Drink a little milk before you go to bed. The small boost of calories will prevent your body from turning to muscle for energy while you sleep, which will slow down your progress of building larger muscles. Have your milk with a bit of cereal, or try yogurt or cottage cheese with fruit.

142.   Measure body fat, not body weight. Do not get discouraged if you are attempting to build muscle and you do not see a change in your weight. You can lose fat while you gain muscle, resulting in a weight that does not change. A better indicator is measuring your body fat. If your weight is holding steady (or even increasing) while your fat levels are dropping - you are gaining muscle.

143.   Be patient. Building muscle is not a quick fix; it takes time before you start seeing muscle development. This can be discouraging and make you want to quit. However, if you are training with the proper technique and doing what you need to do, trust that the results will come on time.

144.   When trying to build muscle mass quickly, smaller is better. Smaller sets with more weight will add muscle more quickly than longer sets. Between 8-12 repetitions for each set is about the ideal. Give your body plenty of rest between workout routines to allow the body to heal. Muscle is built as the muscles heal.

145.   Try doing real stairs instead of the stairs that your gym has. This can help change the perspective that you have for working out, give you an additional amount of motivation, burn more fat, and build more muscle. The additional scenery could also help you workout for a longer period of time.

146.   You should completely exert yourself when performing weight lifting exercises in order to maximize your muscle gain results. Do this by forcing yourself to keep doing one more repetition until you absolutely cannot. This sends a clear signal

to your body that you need more muscle. Remember to get help from a spotter so that you do not suddenly drop the weight when you are finished.

147.   Eat plenty of carbs. If your body runs short on glucose after hard workouts, your body will use muscle tissue for protein and carbohydrates, undoing your hard work. Stay away from low-carb diets, and eat an appropriate amount of carbs given the intensity of your workouts--possibly a couple of grams of carbs per pound of body weight each day.

148.   For quick muscle building, you need to push your muscles to grow. Believe it or not, if you do not push your muscles to increase in size, they won't. By using the overloading principle, you can push your muscles into growing faster. If you are not familiar with the overload principle, it means you need to work out with weights that are greater than your muscles can comfortably handle.

149.   Adequate rest is important to your muscle-building program. Your body can perform the job of recovering from muscle fatigue best when you are resting, so make sure to get at least 8 hours of sleep a night. Failure to do this can even result in serious injury if your body becomes over tired.

150.   Change up your workouts. Research has proven that varying your reps, intensity, and exercises are the best combination for increasing muscle mass. Our bodies are very good at adapting to exercises, and they have to be shocked by changing up the exercises in order to achieve the most optimum growth.

151.   Remember to go to the gym with a friend when you are working on building up your muscles. If you try to do so alone, it is possible that you put yourself into a difficult situation, especially when using free weights. This can lead to serious injuries or lesions.

152.   Before starting your muscle building, you need to sit down and come up with a realistic plan for yourself. This is important because it helps you to follow a set guideline and helps you to reach your goals much faster. If you don't do this, you are likely to give up.

153.   Allow yourself to eat some ice cream. Studies have shown that eating one bowl of any type of ice cream that you like about two hours after a workout does some good. It will trigger the surge of insulin in your body better than many other foods will, and it will taste good too!

154.   Working out can be a very fulfilling experience, but it is one that must be done in an intelligent manner. Never use a new machine or free weight without practicing the proper form first and always be sure to start off with a very low amount of weight as a practice.

155.   One of the most important aspects of muscle building is injury prevention. One of the best ways to avoid lesions and other problems is by warming up before you start your muscle routine. The absolute most important aspect of this is stretching and doing a light cardio routine beforehand.

156.   It is a good idea to work out in the presence of others in order for you to push yourself to your limit. Many people slack off a bit when they are lifting weights if they know that no one is there to notice that they are not working as hard as they could be.

157.   If you want to gain any type of weight during the year, you will need to complement your workout program with a strong diet regimen. This means that you will need to eat more calories in each of your meals. Consume large quantities of meat and potatoes to pack on the protein so that you can be in the best position to gain muscle.

158.   It is important to eat foods and meals with carbohydrates after your workout and on your rest days. This will help you to rebuild and grow your muscles faster. The reason for this is that consuming carbohydrates causes the production of insulin in your body which in turn slows down the rate at which your body breaks down proteins. Even something as simple as a banana or a peanut butter sandwich will help.

159.   Be patient. Building muscle is not a quick fix; it takes time before you start seeing muscle development. This can be discouraging and make you want to quit. However, if you are training with the proper technique and doing what you need to do, trust that the results will come on time.

160.   Don't try to focus on both cardio and strength at the same time. This is not to say you should not perform cardiovascular exercises when you are attempting to build muscle. In fact, cardio is an important part of physical fitness. However, you should not heavily train cardio, such as preparing for a marathon, if you are trying to focus on building muscle. The two types of exercises can conflict, minimizing effectiveness on both fronts.

161.   Are you trying to add muscle mass to your body? If you are eating calorie-dense foods and are

performing muscle build workouts but are still not seeing the results that you desire, you might want to consider adding creatine supplements to boost the growth of your muscles. Creatine aids in building muscle mass. Not only is this supplement popular with many professional bodybuilders, it is also popular with many elite athletes in other sports.

162.   If you have been weight training for a period of time and want to see results a bit more quickly, work on your large groups of muscles, such as those in your legs, back and chest. Some great exercises for those groups are deadlifts, squats, bench presses, dips and military presses.

163.   Set muscle building goals for yourself and evaluate your progress. It can be discouraging to see great muscle bound bodies around the gym, but you have to know that those bodies did not happen overnight. Set specific goals you can reach, and monitor your progress. If you are not seeing the results, you want, you may have to tweak your workouts to get back on the right track.

164.   Talk to your doctor about which supplements are safe for you. You may be able to enhance your muscle building efforts with creatine and other types of supplements, but you need to know if they are healthy for you to take. Taking supplements is

something you need to discuss with a doctor so you can build muscle safely and in a healthy way.

165. In order to build lean muscle you need to work out three to four times per week. You should do workouts that use all the muscles in your body, as this will help you to lose weight quickly and strengthen your muscles at the same time. Working out every day can cause your body to become injured and would be counterproductive.

166. A lot of people believe that they will be able to lose weight strictly through cardio workouts, but muscle building is also very important. It is the best way to boost your weight loss because each pound of fat requires more calories and energy to maintain than a pound of fat.

167. You don't need to get ripped to build muscle. There are many different types of muscle routines, and you must decide what kind you want beforehand. Supplements will need to be added to your diet if you want large muscles.

168. When you first start working out, do not try increasing the weight you are lifting. Instead, work on improving your stamina by doing longer sets or simply more sets. Once working out becomes easier, you can start adding weight or trying harder

exercises to keep your routine interesting and challenging.

169.   Some people have problems increasing all of their muscle groups at similar rates. Fill sets are necessary to pay attention to each muscle group necessary. Fill sets are brief sets of exercises that target the slow-growing group. Do them a few days after the last workout in which the group was strenuously worked.

170.   Calculate your dietary intake to coordinate with muscle building workouts, for faster and better results. On the days you workout, eat well and eat plenty. Taking in the best foods about an hour before your workout will maximize the effects, but make sure not to overeat or consume unhealthy foods as this will be counterproductive to your muscle building efforts.

171.   To help in building lean muscle mass, try mixing up your rep counts. If you normally do 6-8 repetitions, try doing 4-6 repetitions. Your muscles will be forced to adapt in a different way, and you will give your routine a fresh kick. In this way, you will build your lean muscle mass faster.

172.   Focus on one thing at a time. If you want to build mass, you should concentrate on mass

building exercises rather than developing your cardio. Working on your cardio will help you develop other parts of your body and might slow down the building of your muscles if it becomes the focus of your training.

173.   When you are working towards building muscle mass, you have to make sure that you get plenty of sleep every night. If you do not get enough sleep, your body will not build muscle as quickly and there are potential risks for your wellness. Your body needs this sleep to recuperate from the strenuous exercise.

174.   When trying to bulk up and build muscle mass, you should increase the total number of calories that you eat. Eat an additional 3500 calories per week, which will be enough to put on about a pound. Find healthy ways to get anywhere from 250 to 500 more calories daily. If you don't see any weight change, consider altering your eating habits.

175.   As you are lifting weights, do your movements slowly. Moving too fast uses the body's momentum instead of letting the muscles do the work. Likewise, don't swing the weights, because this keeps the isolated muscle from doing the work. This is why going slow seems harder. The isolated muscle is doing its work!

176.   Lifting heavy weights is productive for many parts of the body, but you should avoid lifting extreme amounts of weight when you are working out by performing neck work, dips and split squats. If the exercise puts you in a joint position that is unfavorable, keep the weight limit to a reasonable level.

177.   Many people who wish to build muscle use protein shakes and meal replacements. It is important to note however that there is a distinction between the two. It can be dangerous to your health to use protein shakes frequently as a meal replacement. A full meal contains many essential nutrients that are not included in protein shakes. In addition, living off protein shakes can leave your muscles soft which negates your muscle building efforts.

178.   As you are working to develop muscle, do not count on the scale to tell you how you are doing. You must take the time to measure your body fat to find out how you are doing. If your weight it going up or remaining the same, it may be a sign that you are turning flabby fat into rock hard muscle.

179.   For quick muscle building, you need to push your muscles to grow. Believe it or not, if you do

not push your muscles to increase in size, they won't. By using the overloading principle, you can push your muscles into growing faster. If you are not familiar with the overload principle, it means you need to work out with weights that are greater than your muscles can comfortably handle.

180.   When you're working out for the purpose of building muscle, it's important to consider how much protein you're taking in. The body uses proteins for many things besides building muscle, so if you aren't getting enough, you may not see the muscle growth you want. Make sure to avoid this by eating a diet high in proteins.

181.   When your exercise workout is complete, be sure to engage in a series of stretches to ensure the best environment for your muscles to build and repair themselves. For those who are under 40 years old, they need to hold stretches for at least 30 seconds. If you are over 40, hold the stretch for a minimum of 60 seconds. Stretching properly protects you from injuries related to working out.

182.   Remember that it is never a good idea to use the scale to determine your progress when you are trying to build muscle. If you find that your scale is increasing in numbers, remember that you just might be losing fat while gaining muscle. Since

muscle weighs more than fat, this is a familiar site for many who are trying to do both at the same time. Gauge your results by what you see in the mirror rather than what you see on the scale.

183.   If you are attempting to add some muscle to your body, you should ensure you're consuming an adequate amount of protein. Protein is the primary building block in muscle building, and consuming too little could cause your muscles to diminish, making your efforts in bulking up useless. You may require daily protein in the amount of one gram for each pound you weigh.

184.   Many people overestimate how much protein they need in their diet at the beginning of their muscle building efforts. This can lead to an additional amount of calories than you need, and if you aren't exercising hard, you might gain fat instead of the muscle that you want. Try gradually increasing your protein about three hundred calories every few days so that your body can start building muscle better.

185.   Before starting your muscle building, you need to sit down and come up with a realistic plan for yourself. This is important because it helps you to follow a set guideline and helps you to reach your

goals much faster. If you don't do this, you are likely to give up.

186.   Most people use the same repetition speeds for all their workouts. Try something different the next time you are working out and speed up your repetitions. By using faster lifting speeds, you can actually target and work out diverse muscle fibres, some, which may not get stimulated as often.

187.   Make sure you are getting enough proteins in your diet. You need about one gram of protein for each pound of body weight every day. If you cannot eat enough meat, think about drinking a supplement such as soy milk or even taking a powder supplement. Eating more proteins than you need will not help you build muscles faster.

188.   Vegetables are an essential part of your muscle building nutritional diet. Discussions about good diets for muscle building tend to obsess over complex carbohydrates and proteins; vegetables are largely ignored. Vegetables contain valuable nutrients that are not present in foods that are generally high in protein or carbohydrates. Veggies are also good sources of fiber. Fiber can help the body use the protein more effectively.

189. Do more repetitions, not heavier. The ideal workout to build muscle contains a high number of repetitions at a medium level of intensity. Keep your breaks between sets under a minute. This constant repetition causes a buildup of lactic acid in your muscles, which has been observed to stimulate muscle growth.

190. Animal based products, such as beef and chicken, can help you increase your muscle mass. A good protein target is one gram of protein per pound of mass. When you properly fuel your body with the amount of protein it needs, you help your muscles grow. This can give you the strength and appearance you're looking for.

191. Eating plenty of protein is highly beneficial towards the building of muscles. You can get the mega doses of protein needed for muscle building by drinking protein shakes or taking protein supplements. These are especially effective following a workout or prior to bedtime. Limiting yourself to one shake a day when losing weight is one of your overall fitness goals. In order to bulk up your muscles as well strengthening them, you could consume as many as 3 per day.

192. Only workout your abs muscles two to three times per week. Many people make the mistake of

doing abdominal exercises daily. This does not give the muscles enough time to recover and can ultimately limit their growth and could cause your body to become injured. Working out two to three times per week is sufficient to get lean abs.

193.   If you choose to take any supplements to aide in your muscle building routine, do so cautiously. Many supplements are a complete waste of money, and some can even be harmful to your health. Discuss any of your supplement plans with your physician or a licensed dietician to make sure that you are not harming your body.

194.   Pay attention to your body fat and measure it on a regular basis. Try not to be discouraged if there is not significant weight loss when building muscle, because your weight might not change much using a weight and muscle building routine. Your body fat is a better measure of your overall health as opposed to weight.

195.   On the days after your workouts, it's best to rest and eat a lot of carbohydrates. This helps your body to build muscle and recover from expending energy during the workout. That way, you'll see the biggest muscle growth possible from the workout you did. Pasta, peanut butter sandwiches, and similar foods are great for this.

196.   Carbohydrates are your friend when striving to build muscle mass. When you are exercising hard your body uses significant amounts of carbohydrates fueling your body and keeping you going. If you do not have sufficient carbohydrates to fuel your exercise, your body will break down muscles for protein to keep you going, and you will lose mass.

197.   If you are unsure of what exercises to do more often, throw in more dips, push-ups and chin ups. These exercises have stood the test of time in their proven ability to build upper-body mass. Nor are they likely to be replaced by other possibilities in the near future.

198.   In order to build muscle it is important for you to properly fuel your body. Drinking a protein shake that is loaded with essential vitamins is a great way to give your body the nutrients it needs to repair torn muscle fibers and ultimately build the larger muscles you want.

199.   Pre-exhaust is one method used to help you with muscles that might not quite be strong enough. For instance, your biceps could fatigue before lats on rows. A good fix for this is to do an isolation exercise that doesn't emphasize the bicep muscle,

like straight arm pulldowns. That way when you are working your lats, you are not using the energy of your biceps, and they can get a more effective workout.

200. Use compound exercises to more efficiently add mass to your muscles. Exercises that target a single muscle group are fine later on, but when you are trying to bulk up in general, it's best to hit as many muscle groups as you can simultaneously. Pull-ups, chin-ups, squats, deadlifts and bench presses are all great exercises that work several muscle groups.

201. The "rest pause" method can help you power on to the end of an exercise that challenges you. Simply take a brief break (no more than ten to 20 seconds) in the relaxed part of the exercise. Remain in position and gather the stamina you need to pump out three or four more reps instead of giving up.

202. There are the "big three" when it comes down to the subjects of weight training exercising and building muscles. The main three things to focus on are the squat, the bench press and the dead-lift. Other trainers may call them other names, but they are all essentially the same thing, There three foundations of muscle building are essential because they add bulk and muscle mass, they increase strength and endurance. All muscle-building plans

should include these as an important foundation to build on.

203.   It is important to incorporate a sufficient amount of vegetables into your diet. Most of the muscle building diets ignore vegetables and focus more on proteins as well as complex carbohydrates. Vegetables contain valuable nutrients that are not present in foods that are generally high in protein or carbohydrates. An additional benefit is that these are all great sources of fiber. Your body uses fiber to process protein more efficiently.

204.   If you are trying to build muscle, you are going to have to start eating more over all. Shoot for enough calories in your daily diet to gain a pound per week. Consider the ways you might increase your calories and protein intake, then reconsider your approach if you don't put on any weight in 14 days.

205.   Stay active on your rest days. Being active increases your blood flow, and will help you to recover more quickly. The activity can be as simple as going for a walk. You can also go swimming, biking, or even get a massage. Engaging in these kinds of activities is significantly more effective than simply lying in bed all day.

206.   For quick muscle building, you need to push your muscles to grow. Believe it or not, if you do not push your muscles to increase in size, they won't. By using the overloading principle, you can push your muscles into growing faster. If you are not familiar with the overload principle, it means you need to work out with weights that are greater than your muscles can comfortably handle.

207.   Adequate rest is important to your muscle-building program. Your body can perform the job of recovering from muscle fatigue best when you are resting, so make sure to get at least 8 hours of sleep a night. Failure to do this can even result in serious injury if your body becomes over tired.

208.   It is extremely important that you stand correctly when doing standing exercises, such as overhead presses and squats. These exercises call for a type of athletic stance. In order to achieve this, you should stand with your feet at about the width of your shoulders. Then, slightly point your toes outward, bend the knees, and arch your lower back. Always make sure that your eyes are looking forward.

209.   If your goal is to build muscle, you must increase your protein consumption. Muscle requires protein to rebuild after a workout, and a protein

deficiency will actually reduce your muscle mass. A good measure for your muscle building diet is a gram of protein every day for every pound of your weight.

210.   You need good hydration if you are going to build muscle properly. If you are not drinking enough water, then you can injure your muscles. Hydration is not only important for building muscle mass, but maintaining it as well, so don't neglect this important aspect of bodybuilding.

211.   Developing a smart schedule for your muscle building workouts will keep your muscles growing and keep you from injury. Although a well-conditioned bodybuilder can handle three strenuous workouts in a week, the best practice for people who are just beginning their muscle building is to stick with two sessions per week.

212.   After you have worked out it is important to eat some low-carb protein. This means you probably want to avoid protein bars as they often have high carbs. Good sources of protein include lean cuts of meats and poultry as well as a cheesy omelet completed with some sliced veggies.

213.   Be patient when you are building muscle. Building your muscles properly does take time.

There is no exercise routine or magic supplement that will help you develop your muscles overnight. So be sure to take your time and do it properly in order to keep yourself healthy and help prevent an injury.

214.   When lifting weights, keep your routine on the short side. If you are capable of lifting weights for more than 45 minutes to an hour, then you aren't lifting enough weight with each repetition. Work hard, instead of working long, if you really want to achieve your muscle-building goals.

215.   Make sure your deltoids are fully engaged. By having middle deltoids that are developed, your shoulders are wider and thicker. Make sure lateral raises are above the parallel point in order to get the most out of your deltoid exercises. Begin laterals several inches from the hips in order to decrease the involvement of supporting muscles, such as the supraspinatus.

216.   It's very important that when trying to build muscle you get the proper amount of rest. You need to give your muscles a chance to recover so they can grow bigger. Ideally you want to give the muscles that you just worked on at least 48 hours of rest.

217. When building muscle it is important to be sure that you are giving your body enough fuel throughout the day. You need to up your caloric intake if you want to be able to build muscle and burn as much fat as humanly possible. It is important to learn which foods are best for repairing muscle fibers.

218. Always stretch before you start a workout. Your muscles should be warmed up prior to exercise, in order to avoid injury. Stretching after exercise can help, too, by relaxing your muscles while the start to recover from the workout. It can also be helpful to get massages to relax your muscles.

219. Spread your workouts out so that you are only lifting weights every other day. Spend one day working out your entire body, and then use the next day to rest. Your muscles will grow while you rest, not while you are working out. Even though it might feel like you are doing nothing on your days off, your body is still working hard.

220. When doing weight training, you should always ensure your rest periods are monitored very closely. Short rest periods are the best because they cause a large amount of lactate to accumulate in your muscles. This lactate causes your muscles to be

more fatigued, which can lead to more muscle growth.

221.   Keep in mind that there is no one method to build muscle that will work fast, effectively, and in the area that you really want to target. Muscle building takes work, and it takes time too. If you want to see success you must come up with a solid plan and remain committed to it. Overnight success stories do not happen when it comes to building muscle, so be sure to take it slow.

222.   Mix your weight training up with some high volume intensity and medium volume intensity as well. This means how many reps you do, and also how hard you have to work. Lactic acid will be released while you are working out, and that will stimulate your muscles to grow.

223.   Push yourself hard while you are working out, to the point where you feel like you could not lift one more pound. You want to always be giving your maximum effort if you want to see a payoff. Hard work will equal the results that you are looking for.

224.   Utilize supersets in your workout regimen. By doing two exercises back to back without resting, the working muscles are placed on a much higher demand. Supersets typically include opposing

muscle groups, which include biceps and triceps. By doing an isolation move after a large compound exercise, additional growth can occur.

225.   To build bigger muscles, you should always eat as soon as you get up in the morning. An early breakfast prevents your body from breaking down muscle tissue for energy, which will simply slow down your progress. Choose high-protein foods, and ensure you also eat plenty of carbs at breakfast.

226.   Set short-term and long-term goals. While you should have an idea of what you want to look like eventually, you will only reach that goal by sticking to smaller goals. For instance, try doing just two more bicep curls in your next workout. If you hit a plateau, do not worry. This happens to everyone. Give it time, and you will see progress soon.

227.   It is important for you to wait to do any cardio workout until after you have lifted weights if you are trying to build muscle. Cardio workouts are important for burning calories but they can cause you to push less when you are lifting weights. Lifting weights before doing cardio will help you to be able to truly burn out your muscles.

228.   Mental preparedness is important when trying to build muscle. Before you begin any workout, it is

important for you to be sure you are in the proper mental state to be able to workout. Injuries occur when someone is not focusing on the workout they are doing. Focus is crucial when working out.

229.   When building muscle it is important to be sure that you are giving your body enough fuel throughout the day. You need to up your caloric intake if you want to be able to build muscle and burn as much fat as humanly possible. It is important to learn which foods are best for repairing muscle fibers.

230.   When building muscle, many people make the mistake of over training. When you go to the gym, exercise as hard as possible and take short breaks. Do not do your workouts for more than 60 minutes for best results. Go in, workout, and get out to give your muscles time to recover.

231.   Your body needs fuel for recovery as well as fuel for working out. Consider adding a protein shake to your routine to be taken after your workout. This can be similar to the shakes you already use before exercising, but you can add dextrose to it. Fast-burning carbohydrates like dextrose are okay in this situation, because your energy supplies will be significantly depleted after a good workout.

232.   It is always a temptation to work your reps in each set as quickly as you can, but don't let yourself do it. You will get better results if you do your reps slowly, even if you need to use lighter weights to be able to complete the exercise slowly. Try to shoot for 20 seconds for each rep, with 5-10 seconds for each movement within any weight-lifting exercise.

233.   Technique is the most important aspect of any weight lifting workout. Each individual aspect of your routine needs considerable practice until mastered completely. You should practice early using lighter weights. Once you do this, you can increase your amount of weight and maximize your results.

234.   Regardless of how frequent or intense your workout sessions are, if you are not eating sufficiently, your body will not have enough proteins to build muscle. It is therefore critical to eat meals often. You should strive to consume at least 20 grams of protein every three hours. In addition, it is more important to eat often rather than to eat large portions.

235.   After muscle building workout sessions, be sure to rest well. Many people fail to do this after their workouts, which can be detrimental to their building larger muscle mass. It is when you are

resting that your body grows and repairs itself. If you fail to rest after muscle building workouts, or you cut the rest period short, this over training can prevent your body from becoming larger. As you can see, it is important to refrain from cutting back on rest periods that your body needs.

236.   Stay active on your rest days. Being active increases your blood flow, and will help you to recover more quickly. The activity can be as simple as going for a walk. You can also go swimming, biking, or even get a massage. Engaging in these kinds of activities is significantly more effective than simply lying in bed all day.

237.   You also need lots of carbs when building muscles. Carbs are absolutely critical to provide you the energy you require for working out, and if you are short on them, you will waste your protein on energy instead of building muscle. Consume enough carbohydrates so that you can function and make it through all your workouts.

238.   To maximize your muscle building, avoid heavy amounts of cardiovascular training while you are lifting large amounts of weights. If you are trying to build great muscle mass, cardio workouts can get in the way of that. Blending weights and cardio is ok, but if you are doing one or the other to an extreme

degree, you have to cut down on the other in order to get the results you want.

239.   As you are working to develop muscle, do not count on the scale to tell you how you are doing. You must take the time to measure your body fat to find out how you are doing. If your weight it going up or remaining the same, it may be a sign that you are turning flabby fat into rock hard muscle.

240.   When working out to build your muscles, it is important to know what your limits are. If you are someone who is highly motivated, it is sometimes really easy to push yourself too far. Understand your body and know what it could take. Do not try to compete with someone else especially if they are training at a much higher intensity than you are. You do not want to injure your muscles in the process.

241.   You need to drink at least 4 liters of water every day if you want your muscles to grow. The body needs water to function properly but muscles need water to be able to rebuild after a workout and to grow in size. Drinking water is easy if you carry a water bottle with you everywhere you go.

242.   Change up your workouts. Research has proven that varying your reps, intensity, and exercises are

the best combination for increasing muscle mass. Our bodies are very good at adapting to exercises, and they have to be shocked by changing up the exercises in order to achieve the most optimum growth.

243.   Utilize a power rack in order to prevent a barbell from crushing you while doing a large squat. Lots of squat racks contain pins that can be set below the maximum squatting depth. If you reach failure on a rep, you can just allow the weight to drop onto these safety pins. Therefore, you don't have to worry about lifting more than you are capable of.

244.   Try to do bench presses and squats in the same manner that you do deadlifts, which is from a complete stop. Utilize bench and squat movements in the power rack, and allow the safety bars to be set at a certain point where this bar is at the bottom of these moves. You need to let the bar settle on this point. This helps you to remove any elastic tension, which assists you in increasing your strength.

245.   Good sleep will work well with your muscle-building efforts. Since muscle building and recovery go hand in hand, you need to make certain your body is getting all the rest it needs. No getting

enough sleep or rest can interfere with muscle building results and may even lead to injuries.

246.   Do not overlook the importance of rest in muscle growth. Believe it or not, growth actually occurs during rest, so if you are not getting enough of it, your muscled will not grow or be adequately conditioned. Working out stimulates muscles, and during rest your body gets to work at building the muscles. You need to understand this process and factor rest into your muscle conditioning or building routine.

247.   Pressing through the heels is vital when it comes to performing lunges, deadlifts, and squats. Doing this keeps your weight over the hips, which lets you press additional weight without increasing your chance of injuring your knees. If you discover that your weight is mostly on the balls of the feet, then you should readjust your form.

248.   Don't try to focus on both cardio and strength at the same time. This is not to say you should not perform cardiovascular exercises when you are attempting to build muscle. In fact, cardio is an important part of physical fitness. However, you should not heavily train cardio, such as preparing for a marathon, if you are trying to focus on

building muscle. The two types of exercises can conflict, minimizing effectiveness on both fronts.

249.   When following a lifting routine, try to always workout your abs last. When you train your abs before a large body part, you can decrease your strength and increase your chances of getting injured. This is why you should do your ab workout after your main workout, or you could simply make it a separate workout during a different time.

250.   Don't forget about life outside the gym. While muscle building is a great goal with plenty of benefits, remember that life goes on. Some who try to build muscle seem to forget about other activities; make time for friends and relatives. Even better, invite some of them to the gym with you. A well-rounded life is a happy life, and you will feel better about building muscle if the rest of your life is in place.

251.   Genetics are going to play a role in the amount of muscle building success that you see. If your family has not provided you with the right genetics to have the body that you dream of, you may have to work doubly as hard to see any results. That does not mean it is impossible, it just means more hard work.

252. If you want the best results from weight training and increase your muscle mass, you should strive to train at least three times a week. This should provide sufficient the proper amount of exercise that will stimulate your muscles into a building mode. If you are just starting out, two times a week is sufficient until you become adjusted to the new routine.

253. For quick muscle building, you need to push your muscles to grow. Believe it or not, if you do not push your muscles to increase in size, they won't. By using the overloading principle, you can push your muscles into growing faster. If you are not familiar with the overload principle, it means you need to work out with weights that are greater than your muscles can comfortably handle.

254. It is extremely important that you stand correctly when doing standing exercises, such as overhead presses and squats. These exercises call for a type of athletic stance. In order to achieve this, you should stand with your feet at about the width of your shoulders. Then, slightly point your toes outward, bend the knees, and arch your lower back. Always make sure that your eyes are looking forward.

255.   If you are on a program to build muscle, try losing any excess weight you are carrying first. You must consume fewer calories than you burn. Any activity such as mowing the lawn, bike riding or swimming will create a caloric deficit. As you lose weight, you will begin to see your muscles appear. Then it's time to work them!

256.   Several people mistakenly increase protein intake when building muscle mass. This calorie increase can lead to weight gain if there is not enough exercise. Up your protein intake over time, 100-200 calories every three to four days, to ensure your body can keep up.

257.   Know your limits, and push yourself in an exercise to the point at which you hit that limit. For every set, push yourself to the limit and don't stop until you can't do more. If you must, lower your set length.

258.   Knowing the best basic exercises for muscle building will give you fast track results. Be sure to include squats, dead lifts and bench presses to maximize your use of time and energy. These are the three tip muscle builders that will strengthen and build your muscles. Incorporate them into your regular routine and increase the number of repetitions you do in safe increments.

259.   When you are trying to build muscle to improve your health and fitness, it is essential to recognize that rest is just as important as the exercise in encouraging muscle growth. Muscles need recovery time to repair damage and build new fibers. Working out too frequently or too aggressively can work against you in the long run.

260.   Push yourself hard while you are working out, to the point where you feel like you could not lift one more pound. You want to always be giving your maximum effort if you want to see a payoff. Hard work will equal the results that you are looking for.

261.   Make sure you are getting enough protein, but that it is also coming from good sources. You will ideally consume 1.5g of protein for every kilo of body mass. Fish and lean meats are great sources of healthy protein, although limited servings of red meat can mean creatine, which helps. Protein supplements can be used to get to your target number, but should never replace food.

262.   When you lift weights, your technique has more importance than how much weight you lift, how quickly you do the sets or how often you do them. Every exercise in a weight lifting routine should be practiced thoroughly until you have mastered the

proper form. Make sure to get practice with lighter weight so that maximum results are possible later.

263.   A great way to build muscle is to pay close attention to nutrition, and eat a good amount of protein and carbohydrates. By eating every two hours, and ensuring you get no less than 1.5 grams of protein for each pound of your own weight and no less than 2 grams of carbohydrates per pound. You will have the nutritional tools necessary to build muscle.

264.   Even though you might believe lifting heavy weights is the best method of building muscle, this isn't always the case. Lifting light weight is also very important when it comes to building muscle. Lifting different amounts of weight work different muscle fibers, which can help you ensure that your muscle gain is of higher quality.

265.   Prepare your body for your weight training. You must consume about twenty grams of protein thirty minutes prior to your session. This will amplify the muscle building that takes place as you lift. This is a simple as drinking a couple of glasses of cold milk before you weight train, as well as after.

266.   Many people who wish to build muscle use protein shakes and meal replacements. It is

important to note however that there is a distinction between the two. It can be dangerous to your health to use protein shakes frequently as a meal replacement. A full meal contains many essential nutrients that are not included in protein shakes. In addition, living off protein shakes can leave your muscles soft which negates your muscle building efforts.

267.   Make sure that your diet has enough protein when you are trying to build muscle mass. The maximum amount of protein intake you need is about one gram of protein for every pound of your body weight on a daily basis. Slightly more or less protein does not matter too much, but you do need to intake as much as possible.

268.   Having a smart schedule focused on muscle building workouts will help you grow muscles while keeping you from injury. Although a well-conditioned bodybuilder can handle three strenuous workouts in a week, the best practice for people who are just beginning their muscle building is to stick with two sessions per week.

269.   Watch for scams that promise the ultimate level of success with one exercise. Muscle building requires that you switch up your routine sometimes, and do exercises that will work a variety of muscles.

If all you are doing is working with one machine or on one isolated routine, you will never see the results that you are really looking for.

270.   Make sure you are getting enough protein. The ideal diet for muscle building contains one gram of protein for every pound of your body weight every day. For most people, this can be achieved through diet alone, and protein supplementation is not usually necessary. Supplementing your daily protein consumption beyond this will usually yield no benefit.

271.   Make sure you are getting enough proteins in your diet. You need about one gram of protein for each pound of body weight every day. If you cannot eat enough meat, think about drinking a supplement such as soy milk or even taking a powder supplement. Eating more proteins than you need will not help you build muscles faster.

272.   Mental preparedness is important when trying to build muscle. Before you begin any workout, it is important for you to be sure you are in the proper mental state to be able to workout. Injuries occur when someone is not focusing on the workout they are doing. Focus is crucial when working out.

273. Consider trying out Romanian Deadlifts. Hamstring curls are great for working the hamstrings, but they only utilize movement at a single joint. However, Romanian Deadlifts let you utilize an additional amount of weight, and they work through the entire hamstring muscle, rising into the glute-ham at the origin of the hamstring.

274. It is a good idea to work out in the presence of others in order for you to push yourself to your limit. Many people slack off a bit when they are lifting weights if they know that no one is there to notice that they are not working as hard as they could be.

275. If you desire to build muscle, one of the most important things to consider is a pre-workout meal. This meal should be filled with protein and carbohydrates, which will give you the energy that you need for your workout. Also, foods that contain these nutrients can help to convert fat to muscle as you lift weights.

276. As you are trying to build muscle, the diet you follow should be one that will encourage muscle growth and supply the proper nutrients they need to grow. Just remember to keep a variety to your diet because you don't want to become bored with it, which could lead to making unhealthier decisions.

277.   Find a good workout partner. Ideally, you should find a partner that is as motivated as you are, or even more so. You can motivate each other. It is also advisable to pick a partner with roughly the same strength as you. If you pick stronger or more experienced than you are, you may find yourself getting frustrated.

278.   Although the urge to power through your sets and crank out reps at the maximum speed is very tempting, resist it! Slower repetitions of the exercises yield better results. Don't be afraid to trade off for a lighter weight in order to accomplish more reps. Strive to take your time, and focus your energy on making each rep last for about 20 seconds. This is the best way to make sure that your exercise plan is an effective one.

279.   Train at least three times per week. You need at least three training sessions every week if you want to see significant muscle growth. If you are really new at weight training, this can be reduced to two at the start; however, you should increase the number of sessions per week as soon as you are able. If you already have some experience with strength training, you can add more sessions as well.

280.   If you would like to build more muscle mass, try to do less repetitions of heaver weights. You will need to increase your weight gradually and strive to lift the heaviest that you possibly can for a minimum of five repetitions. When you can life for five repetitions, it is time to increase weights.

281.   Crank up some music. Research has shown that listening to music you love while you are lifting can help you do more reps than not listening to any music at all or not listening to the music that you like. In addition, having headphones can help distract you from having a conversation with others that will defer your workout.

282.   Genetics are going to play a role in the amount of muscle building success that you see. If your family has not provided you with the right genetics to have the body that you dream of, you may have to work doubly as hard to see any results. That does not mean it is impossible, it just means more hard work.

283.   Do not attempt extreme cardio training with weight training. Done within reason, this combo can be truly beneficial for your health, but when done in extreme fashions can contradict one another minimizing the results that you see from

either one of them. Pick one to focus on and stay committed to working on it regularly.

284.   Knowing the number of sets that work for your body is vital for building muscle mass. Many experts recommend you do around twelve to sixteen sets for your large muscle groups, such as your back, chest, and legs, and about nine to twelve sets for your smaller muscle groups, such as your calves, shoulders, and arms. Although this might work for some people, this can cause others to overtrain or undertrain. This is why you must understand the way your body responds to workouts.

285.   Always use your own intuition when working out. Although planning out your workouts ahead is good for making sure that you stay accountable, sometimes you can't always stick to this schedule. For example, you might not be ready for another quad session after your last session left you exhausted. On the other hand, your arms could be well rested after a good workout just a few days ago. Listen to what your body tells you, and follow it.

286.   If you want to build your muscles, the most important thing to do is start a rotation. It is not feasible to work on the same muscle group every day. Doing so is a quick way to ruin your work as well as burn yourself out very quickly at the gym.

287.   It is a common error to drastically raise protein intake immediately upon starting muscle building programs. By doing this, too many calories are being consumed and if a person is only exercising a small amount, fat can increase. Slowly increase protein intake, about 200 calories daily, and you will have a much better chances of building muscle.

288.   When you want to concentrate on building muscle, then you need to realize that what you are eating to aid in muscle growth is almost as important as how you are training those same muscles. If your diet is lacking, then you may just be sabotaging what you can accomplish in your muscle workout.

289.   Squats are perhaps the most important exercise for building muscle mass. Beyond building the leg muscles, squats are an excellent whole-body workout. They work out the arms, chest, abdominal muscles and even the back. Using a proper technique is essential with squats. For a proper squat, the hips should come lower than the knees and the body should remain balanced.

290.   If you wish to bulk up, try to focus on doing bench presses, squatting, and dead lifting. Focusing on these three types of exercises helps build muscle

mass fast. You can add different exercises to your routine, but these three should really be at the core.

291.   Not all supplements are equal when it comes to helping you build the muscles you need. Try to avoid any supplements that have heavier substances. Most professionals recommend using nothing stronger than a basic whey protein so that you don't cause any nasty side effects to your own body.

292.   Utilize giant sets on occasion. A giant set is when you do at least four exercises for a single muscle group simultaneously without resting. Do one or two of these giant sets in order to shock a muscle into growing. For your smaller muscles, which include your shoulders, biceps, and trips, a single giant set is adequate in order to achieve a complete workout.

293.   Consider using strip sets when working out. This involves doing as many reps of a weight as you can, and after doing this, reducing the weight by up to twenty to thirty percent and going to failure again. This method can help you grow those stubborn muscles that just won't grow anymore.

294.   If you have been weight training for a period of time and want to see results a bit more quickly,

work on your large groups of muscles, such as those in your legs, back and chest. Some great exercises for those groups are deadlifts, squats, bench presses, dips and military presses.

295.   If you want to build muscle, give yourself enough time for recovery. It may seem tempting to go full steam ahead, but your body needs time off so you do not hurt yourself. Stick to a muscle-building routine that is about three times a week; beginners may need to start with twice a week.

296.   In order to successfully gain muscle, it is important to have a strategy, and a plan to execute that strategy. There are various resources that you can utilize to determine which strength-training exercises your plan will incorporate. You should also set a schedule that is easy to follow, and will not overwhelm you. Go over your plan with a professional trainer to make certain that it can fulfill your goals.

297.   Try doing real stairs instead of the stairs that your gym has. This can help change the perspective that you have for working out, give you an additional amount of motivation, burn more fat, and build more muscle. The additional scenery could also help you workout for a longer period of time.

298.   Do not attempt extreme cardio training with weight training. Done within reason, this combo can be truly beneficial for your health, but when done in extreme fashions can contradict one another minimizing the results that you see from either one of them. Pick one to focus on and stay committed to working on it regularly.

299.   You need to be focused on what you are striving to achieve when looking to build your muscles. Do not train for endurance and focus on cardio when trying to build muscle mass. Cardio and weight training are a great combination, but they will contradict each other if you have excess cardio in your muscle building routine.

300.   Only workout your abs muscles two to three times per week. Many people make the mistake of doing abdominal exercises daily. This does not give the muscles enough time to recover and can ultimately limit their growth and could cause your body to become injured. Working out two to three times per week is sufficient to get lean abs.

301.   Spread your workouts out so that you are only lifting weights every other day. Spend one day working out your entire body, and then use the next day to rest. Your muscles will grow while you rest,

not while you are working out. Even though it might feel like you are doing nothing on your days off, your body is still working hard.

302.   Remember that it is never a good idea to use the scale to determine your progress when you are trying to build muscle. If you find that your scale is increasing in numbers, remember that you just might be losing fat while gaining muscle. Since muscle weighs more than fat, this is a familiar site for many who are trying to do both at the same time. Gauge your results by what you see in the mirror rather than what you see on the scale.

303.   One problem that can plague a person trying to maximize their muscle-building results is individual muscle groups that grow more slowly than others. Use a fill set when trying to target the problem muscle groups. Completing 25-30 reps of an exercise which targets that muscle group a few days after you've extremely worked it out will increase the visible mass.

304.   Have a protein-rich snack before and after muscle-building workouts. Try taking in 15 grams within a half hour preceding training and 15 grams following the workout. This is equal to consuming approximately a glass or two of milk.

305.   After you have worked out it is important to eat some low-carb protein. This means you probably want to avoid protein bars as they often have high carbs. Good sources of protein include lean cuts of meats and poultry as well as a cheesy omelet completed with some sliced veggies.

306.   Make sure you are getting enough protein. The ideal diet for muscle building contains one gram of protein for every pound of your body weight every day. For most people, this can be achieved through diet alone, and protein supplementation is not usually necessary. Supplementing your daily protein consumption beyond this will usually yield no benefit.

307.   One very important you can do for your muscle building program is to keep a training diary. Keep a log of what kind of exercises you do, the amount of weight you are lifting along with any changes. This way you won't forget your routine and any increases in weight or other changes you have made. Your progress will go forward if you keep track of everything.

308.   You should monitor your intake of carbohydrates. If your diet is too poor in carbs, your muscles will be used to fuel your body while you exercise. You should be eating between two

and three grams of carbs for each pound of your weight every day. Make sure you are getting your carbs from healthy aliments.

309.   When building muscle it is important to be sure that you are giving your body enough fuel throughout the day. You need to up your caloric intake if you want to be able to build muscle and burn as much fat as humanly possible. It is important to learn which foods are best for repairing muscle fibers.